Allen Carr

The illustrated easy way to  stop smoking

Allen Carr

The illustrated easy way to stop smoking

I'M FREE!

This book is dedicated to Afsoon

This edition published in 2017 by Arcturus Publishing Limited
26/27 Bickels Yard, 151–153 Bermondsey Street,
London SE1 3HA, UK

Copyright © 2008, 2014 Allen Carr's Easyway (International) Limited
Illustrations copyright © 2007 Bev Aisbett

AD000036NT

Printed in the UK

ALLEN CARR

Allen Carr was a chain-smoker for over 30 years. In 1983, after countless failed attempts to quit, he went from 100 cigarettes a day to zero without suffering withdrawal pangs, without using willpower, and without putting on weight. He realized that he had discovered what the world had been waiting for – the Easy Way to Stop Smoking, and embarked on a mission to help cure the world's smokers.

As a result of the phenomenal success of his method, he gained an international reputation as the world's leading expert on stopping smoking and his network of clinics now spans the globe. His first book, *Allen Carr's Easy Way to Stop Smoking*, has sold over 12 million copies, remains a global bestseller and has been published in more than 40 different languages. Hundreds of thousands of smokers have successfully quit at Allen Carr's Easyway Clinics where, with a success rate of over 90%, he guarantees you'll find it easy to stop or your money back.

Allen Carr's Easyway method has been successfully applied to a host of issues including weight control, alcohol, and other addictions and fears. A list of Allen Carr clinics appears at the back of this book. Should you require any assistance or if you have any questions, please do not hesitate to contact your nearest clinic.

For more information about Allen Carr's Easyway, please visit
www.allencarr.com

SO YOU WANT TO QUIT SMOKING?

It may seem **OBVIOUS** that,
if you've picked up this book,
you're ready to
QUIT SMOKING!

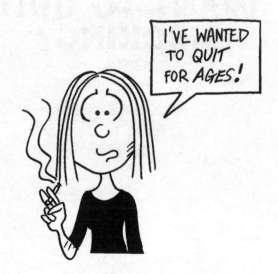

GOOD FOR YOU!
The thing is...are you
PREPARED to quit?

What if I were to say:

'Okay, if you're serious,
STOP SMOKING
RIGHT NOW!'?

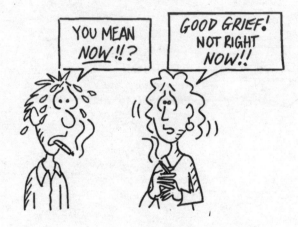

This is a **TYPICAL REACTION** of course.

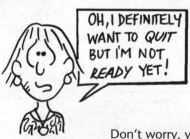

Don't worry, you don't have to quit
until you *ARE* ready.

THE ILLUSTRATED <u>Easyway</u>

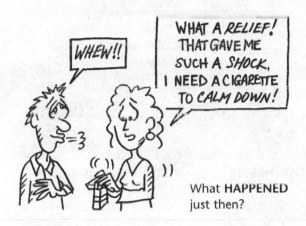

What **HAPPENED**
just then?

What we saw was the terrible **TUG OF WAR**
that smokers go through most of their lives.

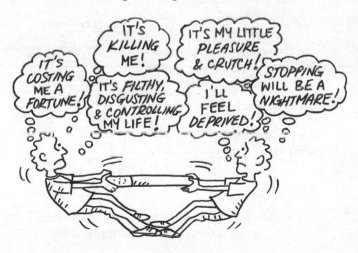

11

You have probably already
tried to quit
MANY, MANY times
using…

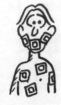

PATCHES

GUM

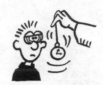

HYPNOSIS

ACUPUNCTURE   or   **COLD TURKEY**

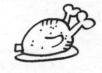

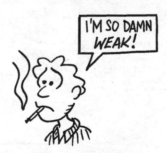

But sooner or later,
sure enough, you're
BACK AT IT AGAIN
and **HATING YOURSELF**
for it.

By now, you have probably become convinced
that you just don't have the **WILLPOWER**.

Actually, it takes a lot of
WILLPOWER
to be a committed
SMOKER.

You need to be able to **PUT UP** with:

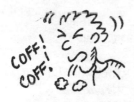

...ILL HEALTH...

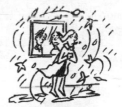

...ISOLATION...

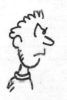

...DISDAIN...

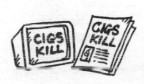

...BAD PRESS...

...COST...   and

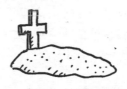

...BLEAK FUTURE
PROSPECTS.

WILLPOWER sets up a **TRICKY DYNAMIC** –
it's called **RESISTANCE**.

Whenever you start **FIGHTING** something,
it tends to get **BIGGER**.

Ever noticed
that if you are **ANNOYED** by something,
it seems to **TURN UP EVERYWHERE**?

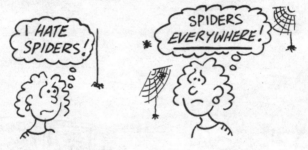

So, of course, what do you think happens when you're
FIGHTING, RESISTING, or are
NOT ALLOWED TO SMOKE?

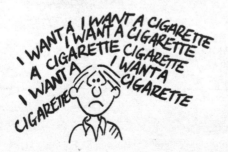

It becomes
*ALL YOU
THINK
ABOUT!*

The more **POWERFUL** the reasons for quitting,
the more **PANICKED** you are likely to
become about *HAVING* to quit!

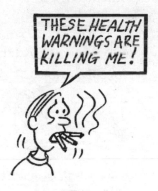

If you're repeatedly
bombarded
with messages of
**DOOM AND
GLOOM,**
what happens?

You feel **STRESSED**
and when stressed,
you reach for your
CRUTCH.

FEAR ⟶ *STRESS* ⟶ *SMOKING*

You want to **QUIT**
but you want to
SMOKE!

You end up at **WAR**
with yourself.

Maybe you didn't feel
READY to quit, but
you feel **PRESSURED**
to do so.

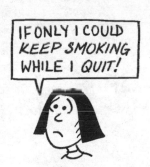

Someone who cares about you may have given you this book in the hope that you might **QUIT**.

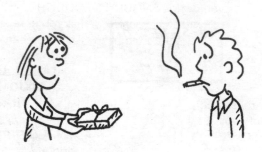

If so, please respect them enough to at least
READ IT.

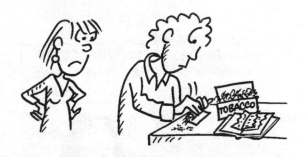

After all, you want to stop anyway and
what **HARM** could it do?

Whatever the motivation –
**HEALTH WORRIES,
COST, APPEASING OTHERS** –
you decide **ENOUGH'S ENOUGH**
and steel yourself to make
a valiant attempt to **QUIT**.

You muster all
of your
RESOLVE...

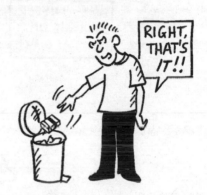

...go **COLD TURKEY**...

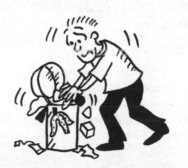

...and
FAIL!!

17

Now, *here's* something to **THINK** about.

When you put out a cigarette,
**YOU ARE ALREADY A
NON-SMOKER...**

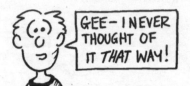

...UNLESS YOU
LIGHT ANOTHER
ONE!

And here's some more
GOOD NEWS.

You are *LESS* likely to
succeed using *WILLPOWER*!

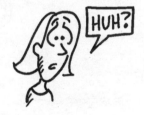

Oh, some people have
succeeded, for sure
(and **GOOD ON THEM**),
but the majority **FAIL**.

In fact, some people have had to exercise that same
WILLPOWER
to fight off the desire to smoke for **YEARS**!

Are they **FREE**?
Not really.

They still **WANT** to smoke and some never get
FREE OF THAT DESIRE.

They continue to feel as though they're
MISSING SOMETHING.
That battle is **EXHAUSTING!**

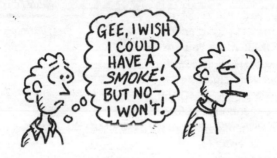

Are these people truly **NON-SMOKERS**
or **SMOKERS** who just aren't **SMOKING?**

There's a **VITAL DIFFERENCE** here
that warrants further exploration.

Q. WHAT'S THE DIFFERENCE BETWEEN A SMOKER AND A NON-SMOKER?

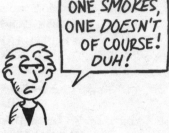

Well, yes...but that could mean that you're only a **SMOKER** when you are actually SMOKING and, in between cigarettes, you are a **NON-SMOKER**, as we mentioned before.

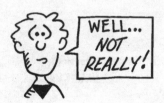

But do you **FEEL** like a **NON-SMOKER** between cigarettes?

So what's the real difference?

GIVE UP?

(Good idea, by the way!)

A. THE NON-SMOKER HAS NO DESIRE TO SMOKE

Given this definition, a person who has 'QUIT' but still yearns for a cigarette is still **HOOKED**!

Not **PHYSICALLY** but **MENTALLY**.

The same goes for **SUBSTITUTES** such as **PATCHES, PILLS** and **POTIONS**. You're still **ATTACHED** to the **ADDICTION** – you're just **SWAPPING** one for another.

Instead of feeling **FREE**, you are driven almost **INSANE** by that constant, nagging thought:

'I WANT A CIGARETTE!'

Eventually, it all gets **TOO HARD** and you give in and **LIGHT UP** that first cigarette...

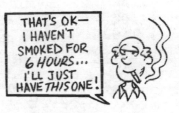

...and then the **NEXT**...

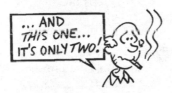

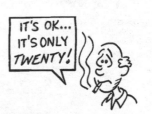

...and then the **REST**!

Being **FREE** means no longer
CRAVING, DESIRING, NEEDING, or **WANTING
A CIGARETTE.**

In order to get to that point,
you'll need to understand what's
REALLY GOING ON.

Every **SMOKER** starts off as a **CASUAL SMOKER.**
We figure that we can **CONTROL** our smoking.

In fact, we don't even **WORRY** about it.

Any problems are way off, in some abstract, distant future.
We think we'll be able to deal with any issues later.

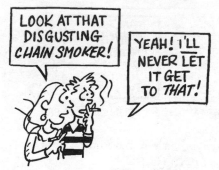

By the time that 'distant future'
becomes the present,
it's *TOO LATE.*

You're **HOOKED.**

So, who's *REALLY* in **CONTROL?**
You've **GUESSED IT!**

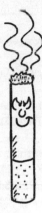

So, if the problems with your smoking are still something
you will deal with in the **FUTURE**,
how will you know when it *IS* time to quit?

When you get:
EMPHYSEMA?   **LUNG CANCER?**

Or you have to have an
AMPUTATION?

How long are you prepared to live in constant **FEAR**
that the next cigarette could be a trigger for **CANCER?**

But you KNOW this stuff ALREADY, don't you?

Well, if so, why haven't you **STOPPED**?

Quite simply, because you can't bear the thought of being without your **PLEASURE** or **CRUTCH**.

And you **CAN'T**, because you are **ADDICTED**.

This isn't designed to scare you – **SHOCK TACTICS** also create **RESISTANCE**.

They just make you bury your head further in the sand.

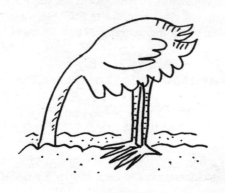

But what we do need to do is

CHANGE YOUR MIND

about your

'BEST BUDDY'!

THE TRAP

Becoming addicted to cigarettes is a bit like falling under a **SPELL**.

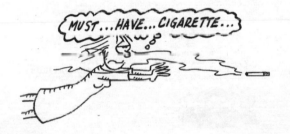

You think that you are in
CONTROL...

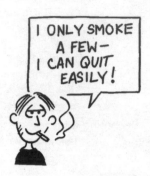

...until you try to **QUIT**.

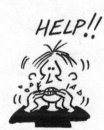

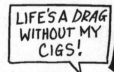

The **ADDICTION** also traps you into
thinking that smoking **GIVES** you
something, and that you
NEED cigarettes to provide
that something.

This trap of addiction is both
POWERFUL and **SUBTLE**.

Let's take a look at how it works
by using the example of the **FLY**
and the **PITCHER PLANT**.

Here is a fly happily
buzzing along.

It doesn't **NEED**
anything to
feel complete –
nature has provided
abundantly to sustain the
fly's existence.

But on this particular day,
the fly happens to
spot an
**UNUSUAL, EXOTIC,
ENTICING BLOOM** and it
gets curious...

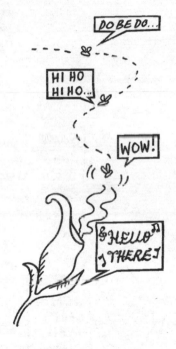

The fly goes **EXPLORING**…

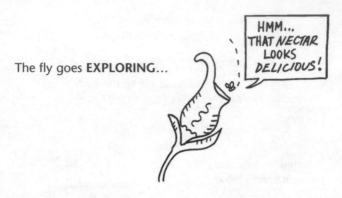

…only to find that this trip is *ONE WAY*.

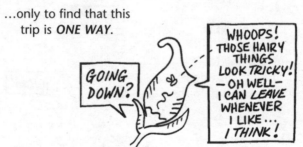

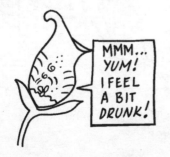

However, the fly isn't particularly **BOTHERED** by this… in fact, he's having a **GRAND OLD TIME!**

But after some time the fly
finds himself getting a bit **FED UP** with this.

What started off as
ENJOYABLE is now making him feel **SICK**...

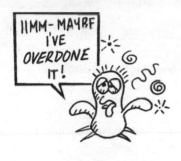

...and it is then it
dawns on him
that something **BAD**
is starting to happen
here...

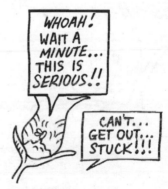

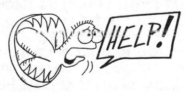

...he realizes that the delicious nectar he was eating before is
now *EATING HIM*!

31

All SMOKERS are like that fly at various stages of descent inside the plant:

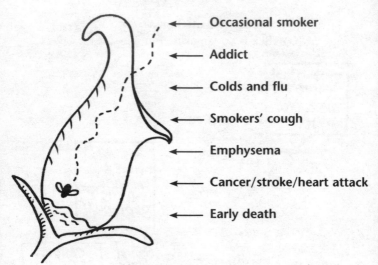

← Occasional smoker

← Addict

← Colds and flu

← Smokers' cough

← Emphysema

← Cancer/stroke/heart attack

← Early death

The most sinister aspect of this trap is that it creates several **ILLUSIONS**:

- **THAT SMOKING IS ENJOYABLE**
- **THAT PEOPLE CHOOSE TO SMOKE**
- **THAT CIGARETTES TASTE GOOD**
- **THAT SMOKING RELIEVES BOREDOM**
- **THAT SMOKING AIDS CONCENTRATION**
- **THAT SMOKING ALLEVIATES STRESS**
- **THAT CASUAL SMOKERS ARE LESS HOOKED THAN HEAVY SMOKERS**

AND...**THAT QUITTING IS DIFFICULT!**

Once you are trapped, you have handed over
your **POWER** to cigarettes.

Smokers do not **CHOOSE** to smoke.

They feel **COMPELLED** to smoke.

They need a **FIX** to ease the discomfort of not having a **FIX**.

Smokers are **DRUG ADDICTS**.

So you don't think you're
an **ADDICT**?

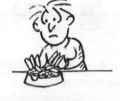

Have you ever smoked
BUTTS?

Have you ever **STOLEN**
someone else's cigarettes?

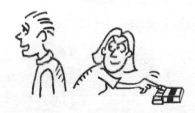

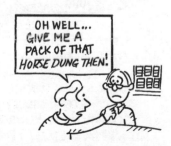

OH WELL...
GIVE ME A
PACK OF THAT
HORSE DUNG THEN!

If you couldn't
get your **BRAND**
would you go **WITHOUT**?

Have you ever **LIED** about how many cigarettes you actually smoke?

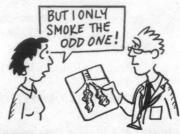

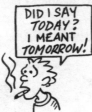

Have you **BROKEN PROMISES** to others (and yourself) that you'll quit?

Have you **PRETENDED** you were out of cigarettes if someone asked you for one?

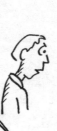

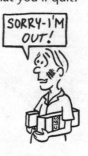

If you ran out, to what **LENGTHS** would you go to get **MORE**?

So, you **STEAL, LIE, CHEAT, HOARD,** and **COMPROMISE YOURSELF** for cigarettes?

Oh yes, you're an **ADDICT.**

ANATOMY OF A NICOTINE ADDICT

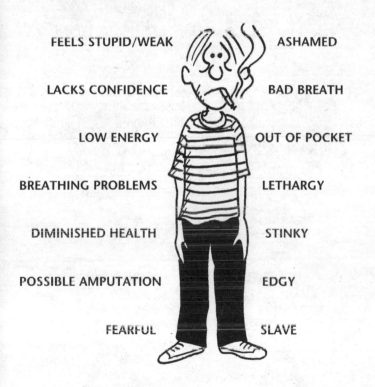

FEELS STUPID/WEAK

LACKS CONFIDENCE

LOW ENERGY

BREATHING PROBLEMS

DIMINISHED HEALTH

POSSIBLE AMPUTATION

FEARFUL

ASHAMED

BAD BREATH

OUT OF POCKET

LETHARGY

STINKY

EDGY

SLAVE

The worst part of being trapped inside the smoking prison is the sense of being constantly pulled in **TOTALLY OPPOSITE** directions.

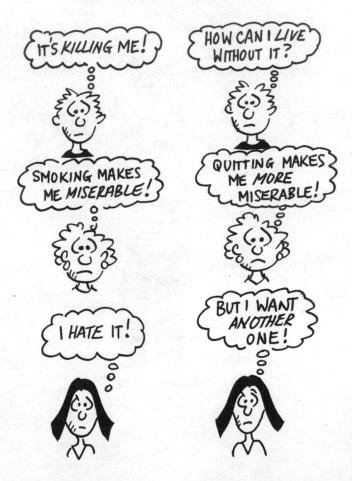

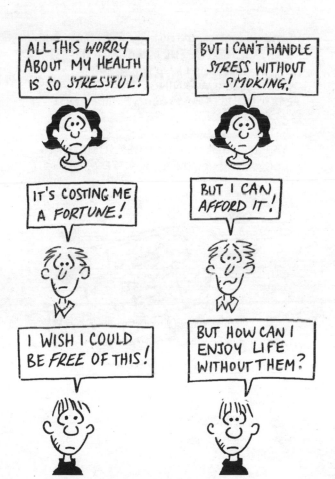

You end up reasoning that there must be something
very **POWERFUL** about cigarettes
that would keep you smoking
despite all the **WARNINGS, HEALTH SCARES,
FEARS, DOUBTS,** and your own desire **NOT TO**.

You think that smoking **DOES SOMETHING**
for you and you think you **NEED** to smoke!

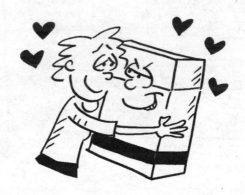

In holding on to such ideas, you have
NO CONTROL
over your smoking.

Instead, you are being controlled by the
SMOKING MONSTER.

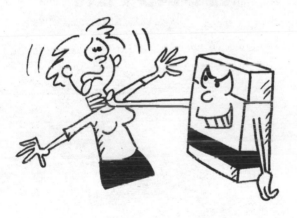

THE
TWO-HEADED
MONSTER

The **SMOKING MONSTER** is **CUNNING**.

It pretends to be your **FRIEND**.

It appears to **HELP** you.

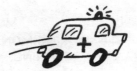

But it makes you think you
CAN'T COPE without it.
Some friend!

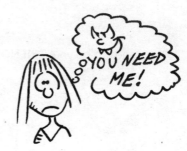

Actually, the **SMOKING MONSTER**
is comprised of **TWO SEPARATE ENTITIES:**

BIG MONSTER and LITTLE MONSTER.

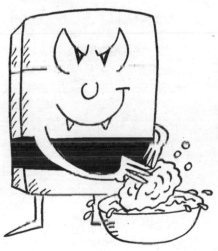

BIG MONSTER
is in charge
of the
BRAINWASHING...

...convincing you that you **NEED** to smoke.

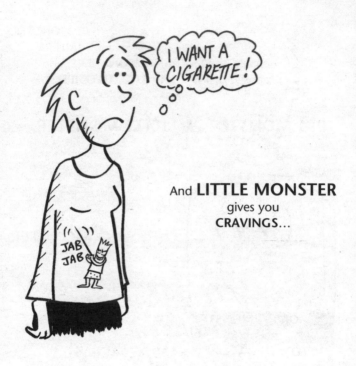

And **LITTLE MONSTER**
gives you
CRAVINGS...

...those **EMPTY, INSECURE** feelings that have
you reaching for a cigarette.

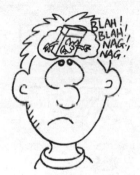

The **SMOKING MONSTERS**
are your **JAILERS**,
OWNERS, and
TORTURERS.

The **SMOKING MONSTERS**
have
TOTAL POWER
over your life.

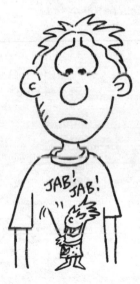

Now, you could be forgiven for thinking that in painting this bleak picture, we are pushing the very **SCARE TACTICS** we said wouldn't work.

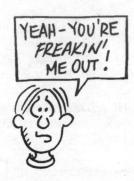

But let's take a look at a couple of things here…

Firstly, these are the **FACTS**, of which most smokers are **PAINFULLY AWARE** (if not, welcome back from **MARS**!).

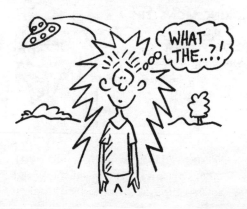

Secondly, despite the **SCARE TACTICS**,
there remains a prevailing attitude
(even among smokers)
that the smoking problem is just a
SILLY HABIT that doesn't warrant
as much concern as other 'hard' drugs.

NICOTINE ADDICTION is rarely referred to as an *ILLNESS* in
the way that **ALCOHOLISM** is.

The view seems to be
that smokers **CHOOSE**
to smoke because they
LIKE it and are simply
being **STUBBORN**
by refusing
to quit.

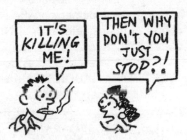

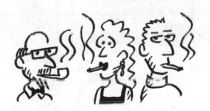

So, the smoker tends to be seen as simply
WEAK, WILFUL, or just plain **STUPID,**
all of which is untrue given the broad
cross-section of society which smokes!

In fact, smokers are just as intelligent and
strong-willed as anyone else.

People who want to get off drugs like
HEROIN or **ALCOHOL**
have far more
PUBLIC RESOURCES
available to them
than the person who wants to kick their
addiction to **NICOTINE**,
which, ironically, is
recognized as being far more
ADDICTIVE than *HEROIN*!

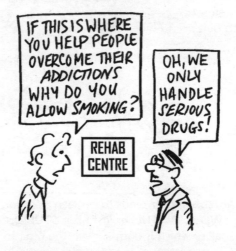

As a result, the poor old smoker who wants to quit has to battle on pretty much **ALONE**, usually with little **SUPPORT**, **SYMPATHY**, or **UNDERSTANDING** of the inner turmoil involved.

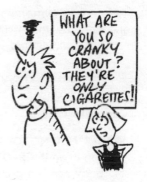

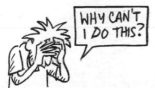

Few non-smokers really understand the genuine **SUFFERING** experienced by a smoker who wants to quit, but can't.

This daily battle with the self can be **OVERWHELMING**.

Smokers trying to quit using **WILLPOWER** can be reduced to tears of shame and despair when, despite numerous **RESOLUTIONS** and heartfelt **PROMISES**, they find themselves unable to break free of the **MONSTER'S** grasp time and time again.

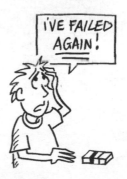

49

Return for the moment to the nicotine addict on p.35 and this time, look with *compassion* at this person who could so easily be **YOU**.

See this person as a **FRIEND** might.

Here is a **CARING, WARM, LOVING, GIVING** person in an **INCREDIBLE** body which represents the pinnacle of creation, but which is trapped in the daily torture of **ADDICTION**.

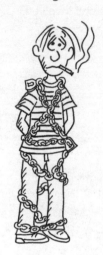

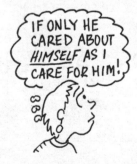

IF ONLY HE CARED ABOUT *HIMSELF* AS I CARE FOR HIM!

Perhaps there might be a greater chance of success if we got rid of the **SHAME** and **GUILT** and started to see ourselves with **KINDER,** more **FORGIVING** eyes.

In fact, it is testimony to the marvels of the **HUMAN BODY** that it is able to cope with nicotine at **ALL**, given that this is one of the deadliest and most addictive substances known, over and above **HEROIN** and **ALCOHOL**.

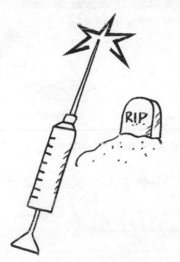

If the nicotine from **JUST ONE CIGARETTE** was injected directly into your vein, It would **KILL** you.

THE GOOD NEWS

is that it takes only a **MATTER OF DAYS** for nicotine to leave your system when you stop smoking and your body **IMMEDIATELY** sets to work to begin repairing the damage.

Once you have freed yourself of the
PSYCHOLOGICAL TRAPS
(the **BIG MONSTER'S BRAINWASHING**),
the **PHYSICAL PANGS** are easy to deal with.

Even **HEAVY SMOKERS** are able to abstain for long periods
without it bothering them while…

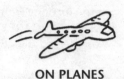

ON PLANES

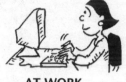

AT WORK

or **DURING A HOSPITAL STAY**.

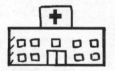

The **PHYSICAL WITHDRAWAL** is not even strong enough to
wake you from sleep.

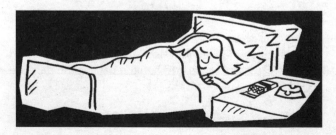

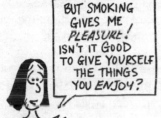

BUT SMOKING GIVES ME *PLEASURE!* ISN'T IT GOOD TO GIVE YOURSELF THE THINGS YOU *ENJOY?*

Sure, but here's something to think about...

SMOKERS DON'T *ENJOY* SMOKING!

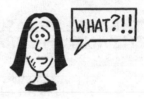

WHAT?!!

I DON'T AGREE! THERE *ARE* TIMES WHEN A CIGARETTE IS *TOTALLY SATISFYING!*

Oh, you mean the *FAVOURITE* cigarettes...

 ...the **FIRST** one of the **DAY**

 ...after a **MEAL** or with a **DRINK**...

 ...after **EXERCISE**...

...and during **BREAKS**...

What these cigarettes have in common is that some time has usually elapsed since you had your last fix and the relief seems all the more precious.

You associate that level of relief with the situation you're in, which reinforces the **BRAINWASHING**.

In the end, you can't enjoy these situations without smoking.

THE SOLE 'PLEASURE' OF SMOKING IS RELIEVING THE CRAVING FOR NICOTINE.

Let's take a look at this:
THIS IS A WELLBEING METER...

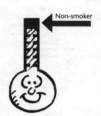

Non-smoker

...this is the level of your **WELLBEING** on a good day before you started smoking.

Then, you light your first cigarette and the **LITTLE MONSTER** is born.

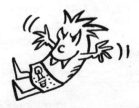

54

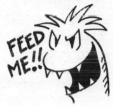

THE LITTLE MONSTER
has a **HUGE APPETITE**
and very soon he demands to be **FED** again...

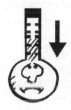

...and your **WELLBEING** drops as you feel that **EMPTY, INSECURE** feeling of the body's reaction to **NICOTINE WITHDRAWAL**...

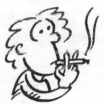

...so you **FEED** the monster again.

There *is* some **RELIEF**...

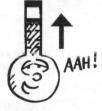

AAH!

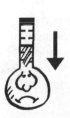

...until the monster gets hungry again!

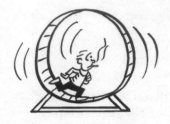

And so it goes...
ON and **ON** and **ON**...

Over time, the body builds up a tolerance to the drug, so that when you smoke it only **PARTIALLY** relieves the feeling, so you feel **MORE STRESSED, MORE OFTEN** and need to **SMOKE MORE**.

No matter how much you feed the **LITTLE MONSTER,** you can *never* reach the level of **WELLBEING** that you felt before you smoked.

Even at your best, you will always feel
MORE STRESSED AND LESS RELAXED
than a non-smoker.

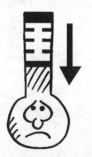

In fact, progressively declining **HEALTH,** feelings of **SHAME, DISGUST,** and **SLAVERY** and the **CONSTANT FEAR** of disease or death looming in the background, ensure that your feeling of wellbeing keeps getting **LOWER** and **LOWER**.

STILL not convinced that smoking is not **ENJOYABLE**?

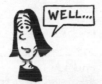

OK. Light one up right now and **INHALE DEEPLY** six times.

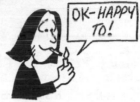

Now, describe the **PLEASURE** you're experiencing.

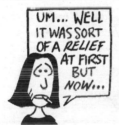

Have **ANOTHER ONE**.

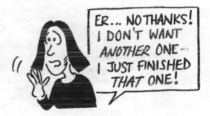

Why not, if it's as **PLEASURABLE** as you say?

It's not about **PLEASURE**.
It's about **TOPPING UP** your **NICOTINE LEVEL** to try to make up for the **WITHDRAWAL** caused by the last cigarette.

You can't **HELP** it!

You need

HELP!

It's OK – **HELP IS AT HAND!**

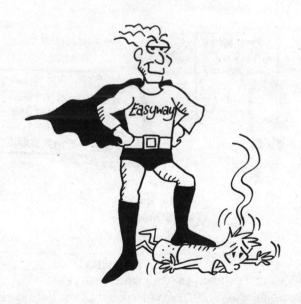

You need to start

CARING ABOUT YOURSELF

enough to

HELP YOURSELF

by working your way,

STEP BY STEP,

through the rest of this book.

NO BUTTS

IMPORTANT NOTE:

YOU CAN KEEP SMOKING
UNTIL YOU 'GET IT'!

IN FACT, WE INSIST
THAT YOU DO.

AS LONG AS YOU STILL
SEE A CIGARETTE AS
DESIRABLE, YOU'LL
BE A SMOKER.

DON'T WORRY –
FOLLOW EVERYTHING
IN THE BOOK AND

YOU'LL GET IT!

Our work begins by taking
a **GOOD, HARD** look
at the monster and
seeing what it
REALLY is...

AN ILLUSION!

It's a bit like the childhood 'Monster-Under-the-Bed'.
Remember how **BIG** and **SCARY** that monster seemed to be
as you lay there in the dark?

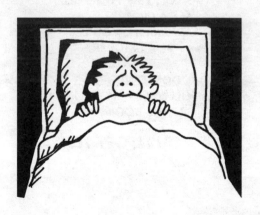

That is, until the time when you finally
screwed up the courage to **LEAN OVER**
to take a **PEEK**...

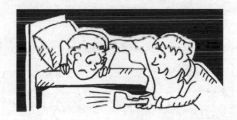

...and all you found there was a
whole lot of **DUST BUNNIES**!

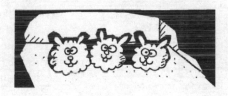

The monster existed only in your
IMAGINATION.

In a similar way, the **BIG SMOKING MONSTER**
feeds on your **FEAR**.

It **BRAINWASHES** you into thinking that you'll be
WORSE OFF without it.

It's time to start shattering some of those **ILLUSIONS**.

 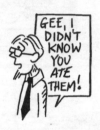

That you like the taste is a
genuine illusion.
All you need to do is
remember how **BAD**
cigarettes tasted when you
first began smoking.

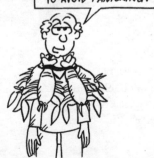

They only 'taste' good
because you are satisfying
the craving for nicotine
and you associate the taste
with relief from the
CRAVING.

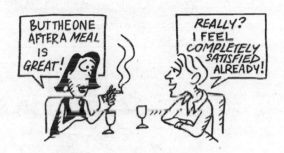

The cigarette after the meal **SEEMS** to taste
better because you're satisfying **THREE** aggravations –
HUNGER, THIRST, and your need for a
NICOTINE FIX.

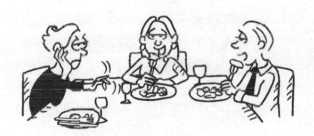

Think of how **FRUSTRATED** you get
when non-smokers are slow at finishing their meal
and you're itching to **LIGHT UP!**

Why would **ONE CIGARETTE**
out of the **SAME PACKET**
taste better than the others?

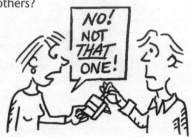

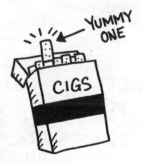

Smoking doesn't improve the taste of food.

On the contrary, it
KILLS OFF YOUR TASTE BUDS.

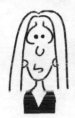

BUT I'M AFRAID THAT IF I QUIT I'LL PUT ON *WEIGHT!*

Weight gain will only be a problem if you **SUBSTITUTE** one **CRAVING** for another.

The point is to realize that you're not **MISSING** anything!

In fact, you'll regain lots of **ENERGY** and be **MORE ACTIVE**. Once your poor old body has been purged of all that **GLOOP**, you'll feel more **ENERGETIC**.

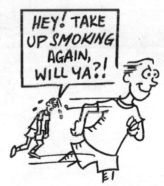

HEY! TAKE UP *SMOKING* AGAIN, WILL YA?!

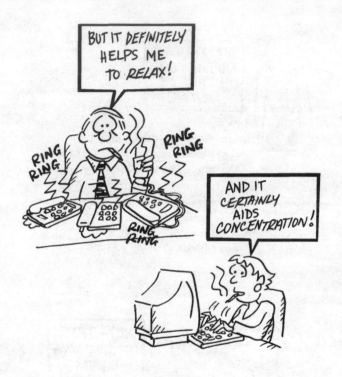

These are two of the most commonly held
ILLUSIONS
about smoking.

Let's shatter them!

To puncture the illusion that cigarettes help you to **RELAX**, imagine that you and a non-smoker are both off to the dentist this morning – an experience that causes most people to feel **TENSE**.

You are already under par because you've woken up with the **STRESS** of having to top up your **NICOTINE LEVEL** which has dropped overnight.

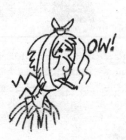

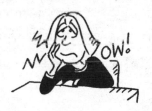

The non-smoker only has to deal with the stress of the **DENTAL APPOINTMENT**.

Now, let's **FAST FORWARD** to the end of the appointment.

You can both heave a big sigh of **RELIEF**...
or *CAN YOU?*

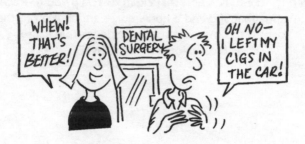

The **REAL** stress for the smoker is in constantly having to
satisfy that incessant **HUNGER**, that **ITCH**,
when the nicotine level drops. This is why it **SEEMS**
that smoking also aids **CONCENTRATION**.

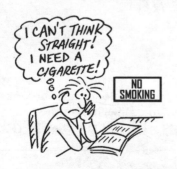

Of course it's difficult to
concentrate when you're
DISTRACTED by the
body suffering from
nicotine withdrawal and the
mind asking for a cigarette.

Non-smokers don't have this problem and nor will you once
YOU ARE FREE!

You experience

MORE STRESS AND A

LACK OF CONCENTRATION

BECAUSE

YOU SMOKE!

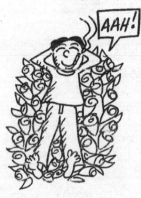

If smoking was the cure-all for stress, your life should be a *BED OF ROSES*.

Non-smokers may experience the same degree of **LIFE STRESSES** as you, but they don't have the **EXTRA BURDEN** of smoking as well.

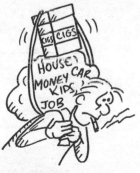

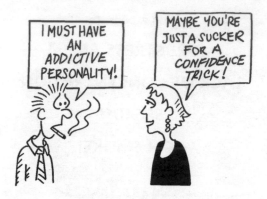

You weren't addicted to your first cigarette.
You had to **WORK** at it.

Think about it, in 1948 in the UK 82% of the male
population were smokers. Today it's less than 20%. Are you
seriously suggesting that in 1948 82% of men had addictive
personalities and now it's down to under 20%?

It's the **DRUG** that addicts you, not your **PERSONALITY**.

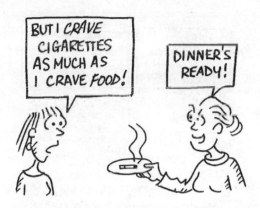

Eating is a **NATURAL** act. Smoking is not.
You are not born with an in-built **TRIGGER**
to smoke, in the same way that
hunger alerts you to **EAT**.

That trigger is **CREATED** by **SMOKING**.

EATING *SATISFIES* HUNGER.

SMOKING *CREATES* HUNGER...

and the hunger that smoking creates is

NEVER, *EVER* SATISFIED!

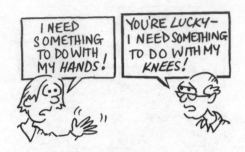

If it's really about needing to keep your
HANDS busy, why **LIGHT UP**?
Why not just handle an **UNLIT** cigarette?

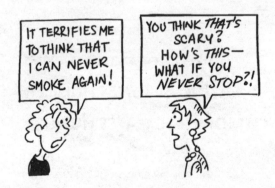

Would it send you into a **PANIC** if you
could never eat **BLACK FOREST GATEAU** again?

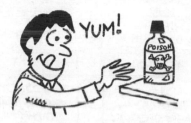

Why should it bother you not to
take **POISON** every day?

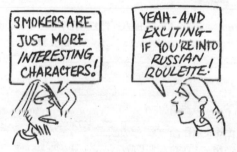

Oh yes, smokers are infinitely more *INTERESTING*
than **BORING, DO-GOODER HEALTH NUTS**.
That **COUGH** alone certainly gets you **NOTICED**!

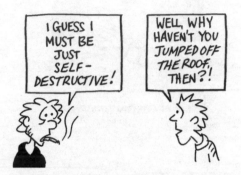

If you're really **SELF-DESTRUCTIVE**, why continue an activity you think makes you feel **BETTER**?

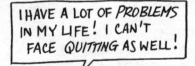

Does **SMOKING** make the problems **DISAPPEAR**?

BUT *SMOKING* IS ONE OF LIFE'S *PLEASURES*— LIKE GOOD WINE & CHOCOLATE! WHAT'S ALL THE *FUSS?*

Would you encourage your **KIDS** to smoke?

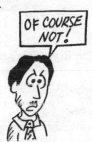

OF COURSE *NOT!*

If you had your life over, would you **CHOOSE** to be a smoker?

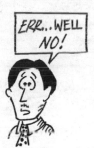

ERR..WELL *NO!*

If it's not a **PROBLEM** and it's so **PLEASURABLE**, why wouldn't you *RECOMMEND* it?

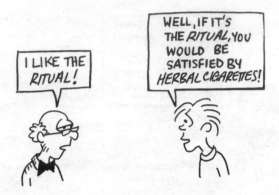

The **RITUAL** is just what you need to go through to get the nicotine into your body.

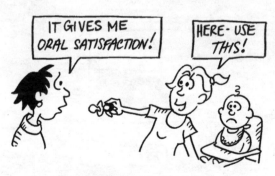

If it's *ORAL* **GRATIFICATION**,
why
LIGHT IT or *INHALE*?

You managed for many years after you were **WEANED**
without needing to stick
a cigarette in your mouth.

Would you walk around sucking a **DUMMY**?

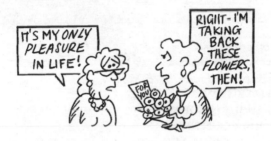

Oh, *COME ON*! What about **FRIENDSHIP, FAMILY,
SUNSHINE, FOOD,
FREEDOM, HEALTH,
HOLIDAYS, NATURE...ETC ETC**?

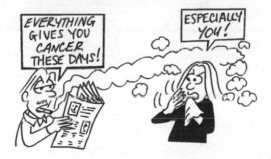

So you picked a **TOP-SHELF CARCINOGEN**!
You must be a **CONNOISSEUR**!

THE ILLUSTRATED Easyway

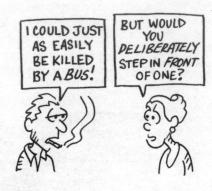

You could also
win the **LOTTERY**,
be discovered for
TELEVISION,
or be elected **LEADER
OF YOUR COUNTRY!**

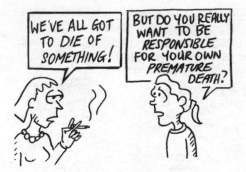

Smoking is **SLOW SUICIDE**.

Besides, do you want the lead-up
to your death to be a
PROLONGED, HIDEOUS TORTURE?

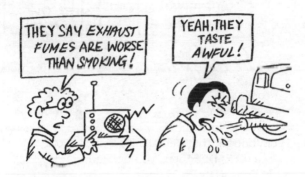

Well, if you're **DUMB** enough to
suck on something **DEADLY**…

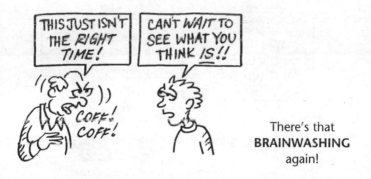

There's that
BRAINWASHING
again!

It convinces you that the time is **NEVER** right!

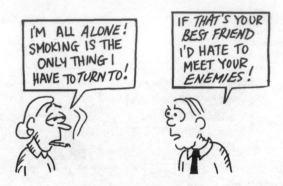

Have you thought that perhaps it's actually your *SMOKING* that keeps you isolated?

And what kind of **FRIEND** would **POISON, CHOKE,** and **IMPRISON** you?

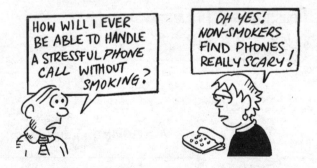

Is the phone about to **BLOW UP? BITE YOU?**
It's the **SMOKING** that's creating the stress.

Can you see how **LAME** these excuses are?

How much of your thinking has been distorted
by the **SMOKING MONSTER'S**

BRAINWASHING?

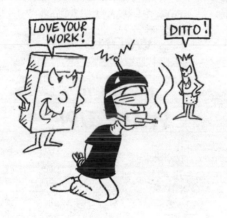

It **CLOSES YOUR MIND**.
It makes you **DEAF, DUMB,** and **BLIND**.

It's part of the **TRICK,** the **SPELL,** the **SMOKESCREEN**.

The biggest **STUMBLING BLOCKS** are the ideas that:

(A) YOU ARE ACTUALLY *SACRIFICING* something.

WRONG!

(B) YOU'LL BE ABLE TO SMOKE OCCASIONALLY AND BE IN CONTROL.

WRONG!

IT'S TIME TO

WAKE UP!

Just for a moment see yourself as a
NON-SMOKER sees you...

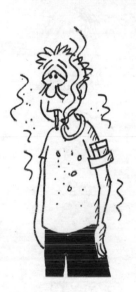

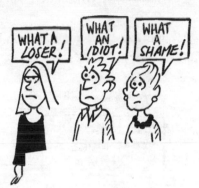

...and ask yourself,
what's so **GREAT** about
smoking that makes you
hang on to it so fiercely?

Could you ever really convince a non-smoker
that you are **BETTER OFF** smoking
than they are **NOT SMOKING**?

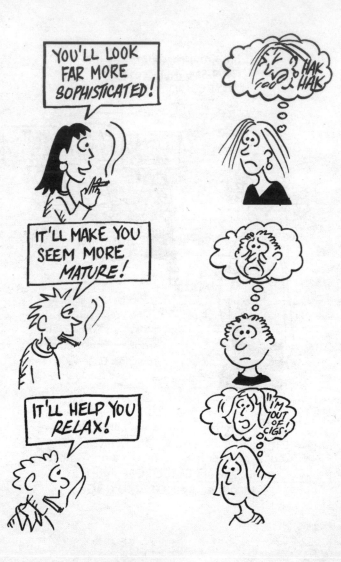

You are being **DUPED** by the
greatest **CON ARTISTS**
of all...

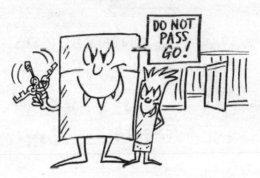

Your JAILERS.

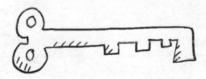

EASYWAY holds the key that will set you free
and it opens only *ONE THING...*

YOUR MIND!

Take off the

ROSE-TINTED GLASSES!

How do you make sure you

NEVER

CRAVE a cigarette?

Remember the **REALITY** of smoking:

IT'S NOT PLEASANT.

IT'S NOT FUN.

IT DOESN'T RELAX YOU – IT MAKES YOU UPTIGHT.

IT CAUSES THE STRESS YOU THINK IT'S RELIEVING.

IT DOESN'T RELIEVE BOREDOM, JUST THE OPPOSITE.

IT DOESN'T HELP YOU RELAX, IT DISTRACTS YOU.

YOU'LL HANDLE STRESS BETTER AS A NON-SMOKER.

YOU'LL ENJOY SOCIAL OCCASIONS MORE AS A
NON-SMOKER.

THERE'S NOTHING TO GIVE UP!

THE JOYS OF SMOKING:

FURRY TONGUE

FOUL BREATH

SALLOW SICKLY COMPLEXION

ENDLESS COUGHING

YELLOW TEETH

LOST MONEY

SHAME & GUILT

FEELING EXHAUSTED

SLAVERY

BAD HEALTH

WHAT IS THERE TO MISS?

We've covered most of the **EXCUSES,**
but there's one more thing that warrants a
SPECIAL EXAMINATION…

FEAR.

THE VOID

The **SMOKING MONSTERS** thrive on **FEAR**.
Of course, this fear surfaces most when
we consider **QUITTING**.

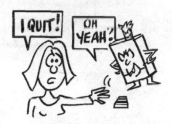

What you need to
remember is
this fear
was
CREATED
BY THE
ADDICTION!

If you are still having **DOUBTS**,
it may be because of this **FEAR**.

Let's begin to **BLOW IT TO SMITHEREENS!**

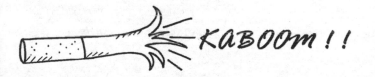

KABOOM!!

A FEAR OF FAILING may be fuelled by focusing on the idea that you are making a **SACRIFICE** or that quitting is something you must **ENDURE**.

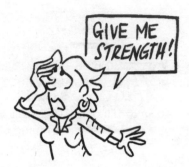

OPEN YOUR MIND!

There is **NOTHING** to **GIVE UP**!

Life is infinitely **BETTER** without smoking!

See quitting as a *REWARD*, not an **ORDEAL**!

But even if you fail, are you any **WORSE OFF** than if you just kept smoking? At least give it a **GO**!

DO NOT DEPRIVE YOURSELF OF THE CHANCE TO BE FREE!

Again, you'll only **STRUGGLE** if you think you're **LOSING** something of **VALUE**!

STOPPING IS NOT PUNISHMENT!

SMOKING IS THE PUNISHMENT!

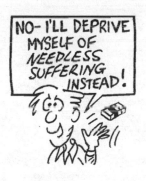

You are about to receive the
**GREATEST REWARD –
YOUR FREEDOM.**

REJOICE!

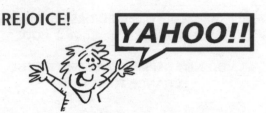

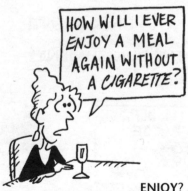

ENJOY? Are you kidding?
You'll finally be able to **TASTE** it!

SAVOUR it!
Now you can **AFFORD** it, order the very **BEST**!

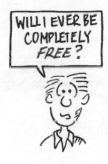

Well, now you're **INFORMED**,
you have **CHOICE**.
That's **FREEDOM**.

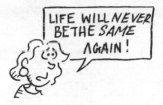

And **HALLELUJAH** for that! **NOW** you have a chance
to really **ENJOY** life.

Of course, you can always
CHOOSE to hand the keys back to your **JAILER**.

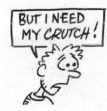
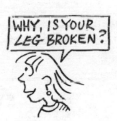

At least you're being **HONEST** about your *ADDICTION*.

Look, you *NEED* **AIR, WATER,** and **FOOD**
for your *SURVIVAL*.

Smoking isn't a **NEED**. It isn't a **CRUTCH**.

It's a **TRAP**.

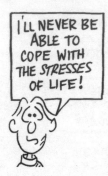

Animals in the wild face **STRESS** every time they are in the vicinity of predators.

They don't need **DRUGS** to cope.

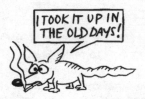

Children don't need **DRUGS**.
They're **HIGH** on life!

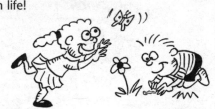

So why do you think we turn to **DRUGS** to feel **OK**?

Because we feel
INCOMPLETE.

You didn't get hooked because you are **STUPID** – and neither are today's young smokers, who are extremely well informed about the **HAZARDS** of smoking!

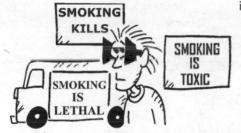

The reasons for starting smoking are still very much about wanting to **FIT IN,** to **BE COOL,** or to **PROVE ONESELF** to **OTHERS** in some way.

Of course, the underlying **BELIEF** behind this is:

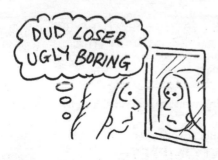

I AM INCOMPLETE

AS

I AM.

In other words, I need some **CRUTCH**, **PROP**, **MASK**, or
ARMOUR to **COMPLETE** me
or **HIDE** my **INSECURITY**.

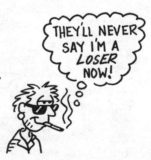

This arises because
we mistakenly believe
that **OTHERS**
have something we lack –
**STYLE, POWER, BEAUTY,
COOLNESS** etc.

So, we **IMITATE**
those we envy or
OUTDO them in terms of
RISK-TAKING or **DARING**,
thinking that we will be
more **APPRECIATED** or
RESPECTED.

Think about those people you thought you needed to **IMPRESS**.

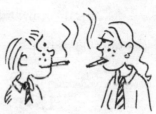

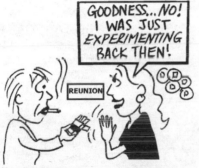

How many are **STILL** smoking?

If you're still needing that **PROP** to cope with feelings of **INADEQUACY**, **STRESS**, or **HELPLESSNESS**, you are still labouring under the **ILLUSION** that you, yourself, are **NOT ENOUGH**.

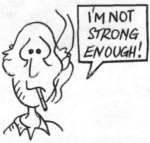

Does **SMOKING** make you feel **BETTER** about **YOURSELF**?

Are you **PROUD** that you smoke?

Has smoking made you feel more **ADEQUATE**?

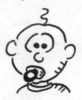

Surely you realize that whatever the reasons were that caused you to start smoking, they no longer apply.

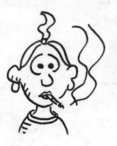

If you're really **HONEST**, you'll admit that you wish you'd never started. Nor can you explain why you continue to smoke.

And here's the **GREATEST IRONY**: you keep topping up the drug in order to **TEMPORARILY** feel the way a **NON-SMOKER** feels **ALL** the time!

The only reason you **LIGHT UP** is to get rid of the feeling of **NICOTINE WITHDRAWAL** which **NON-SMOKERS** do not suffer from in the first place!

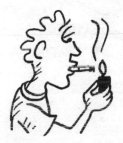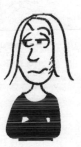

The cigarette does not **RELIEVE** the empty feeling
– it **CAUSES** it!

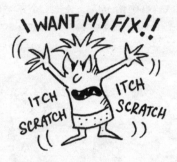

In fact, when you
light a cigarette,
you are trying to feel the
way you did when
YOU were a **NON-SMOKER**.

THOSE TERRIBLE CRAVINGS

By now, you're probably itching to get on with it,
but there's one **LAST THING** we need to take a look at:
those so-called

'TERRIBLE CRAVINGS'.

This has been the little monster's tool to keep you hooked –
that **NAGGING, EMPTY, INSECURE** feeling
that has had you reaching for a cigarette.

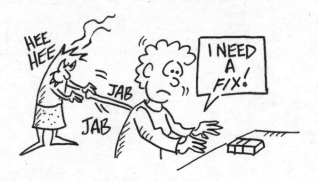

If you really have **GOT IT**,
you will be very clear that these
cravings are mostly **MENTAL**.
If your **THINKING** is right, you're ready to follow the
instructions that will enable you to become a
HAPPY NON-SMOKER.

The biggest part of the job is **ALREADY DONE**.

Once you have the right **MIND-SET**, the **PHYSICAL** cravings are a **MINOR** part of the whole thing.

Even though they are **MINOR**, you will still benefit from having a few **STRATEGIES** for effectively dealing with the **LITTLE MONSTER** while he goes through his **FINAL DEATH THROES** in the first few days.

After all, he's about to be

STARVED!

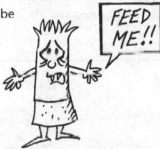

He may not be happy about this, of course. But *YOU* **SHOULD BE**!

Why would you **MOPE** about the death of a *SADISTIC TYRANT*?

Shouldn't this be cause for

CELEBRATION?

NOTHING *BAD* IS HAPPENING!

The **PHYSICAL SENSATIONS** are only slight and will pass in a few days.

Regard any **COMPLAINT** from the monster as a sign that, at last, your **JAILER** is *DYING*, the door is open and you are now **FREE**!

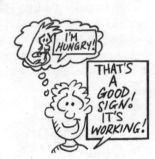

REJOICE!

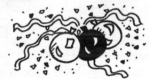

OK then, go on and **THINK** about it! (Remember – what you resist **PERSISTS**.)

But **DO** think about it the **RIGHT WAY**.
Instead of thinking:
'I want a cigarette, but *CAN'T HAVE ONE*',
think: 'Isn't it great!
I DON'T NEED TO SMOKE any more!'

If you have woken up to the **BRAINWASHING**, you have
already **KILLED OFF** the **BIG MONSTER**.
Now, you need only take on his little **PARTNER**.

HANDLING THE LITTLE MONSTER

It's easy! There's no physical pain,
just an occasional '**EMPTY PANG**'.

When this comes, don't think of it as
'I want a cigarette',
instead recognize it as the **LITTLE MONSTER**
demanding its fix, and enjoy
STARVING IT TO DEATH.

In just a few days, you'll never have
to experience it again!

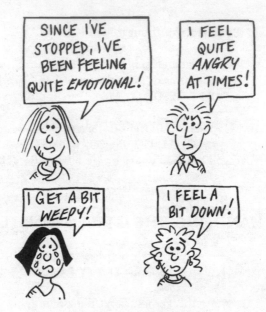

Those emotions were there
ANYWAY.

If this happens, don't worry. Any big change
can be unsettling.

Ask yourself:
What am I really **ANGRY** about?
What do I really feel **NERVOUS** about?
What is the **GAP** in my life that I've used smoking to fill?

Then **ATTEND** to those needs.
They've just been **HIGHLIGHTED** so that you can
HEAL them.

Ask yourself, what started your **SMOKING**?

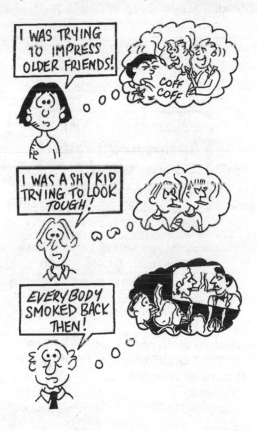

And did **SMOKING REALLY** help you feel more **GROWN UP, PEACEFUL, LESS ANGRY, COOLER,** or **BRAVE?**

DID IT MAKE YOU LESS STRESSED? DO YOU STILL ADMIRE ROLE MODELS BECAUSE THEY SMOKE?

DID SMOKING MAKE YOU FEEL BETTER OR WORSE ABOUT YOURSELF?

THERE'S A SAYING:

> *I am not what happened to me. I am what I chose to become.*

OK. So you made a **DUMB CHOICE** back then
for some pretty **DUMB** reasons...
(most people make several in a lifetime)

...but you now have the opportunity
to make the **BEST DECISION**
you will ever make – one which
you will be **PROUD** of
for the rest of your life...

YOU DON'T EVEN HAVE TO DO ANYTHING.

– SIMPLY DON'T LIGHT THE NEXT CIGARETTE!

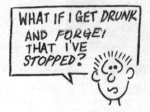

Don't worry. You'll remember before you actually light up and when you do remember, **DON'T MOPE** but **REJOICE** in the fact that you're now **FREE!**

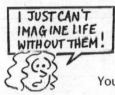

You don't have to **IMAGINE** it.

HERE'S WHAT IT WILL BE LIKE:

You'll have **ENERGY TO BURN**.

You'll **SLEEP BETTER**.

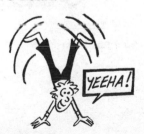

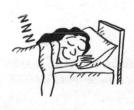

No more **FIDGETING** through a movie or a meal,
HANGING ON for a cigarette.

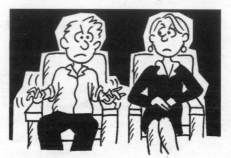

You'll **SMELL FRESH!**

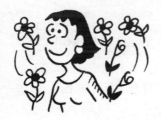

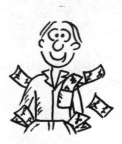

You'll have **HEAPS MORE MONEY**.

And you'll **FEEL SORRY**
for those who **SMOKE**.

Can you picture future historians trying to make **SENSE** of this ridiculous thing called **SMOKING**?

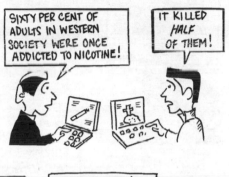

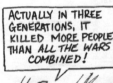

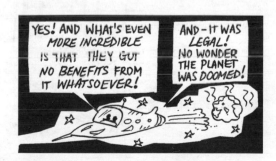

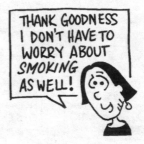

SOONER OR LATER, you'll find yourself going through a challenging experience **WITHOUT** needing to smoke!

The reward is the feeling of **RELIEF** that you're **FREE.**

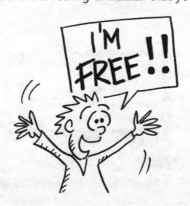

What does smoking do for you?

ABSOLUTELY NOTHING!

What does smoking take from you?

ABSOLUTELY EVERYTHING!

A truly wonderful thing is about to happen –

YOU ARE ABOUT TO RECLAIM

YOUR FREEDOM

AND

YOUR LIFE!

FINAL
INSTRUCTIONS

STOP!

BEFORE YOU READ ON.

If you've **GOT IT**, but feel a little apprehensive,
that's OK. The 'proof of the pudding is in the eating'
as the saying goes.

BUT IF YOU STILL THINK:

• Smoking gives you any **RELIEF**

• You'll keep some cigarettes around 'just in case'

• That you're making some kind of **'SACRIFICE'**

• Just **ONE** now and then won't hurt

• That you can **CONTROL** your smoking

• There's something **POSITIVE** in smoking

• You'll be less **HAPPY, PEACEFUL,** or **FREE** without smoking...

YOU'RE NOT READY.

GO BACK AND READ THE BOOK AGAIN.

MAKE NOTES.

OPEN YOUR MIND!

Soon, you will be smoking the
VERY LAST CIGARETTE
that you will **EVER** smoke in your life.

This will be done with
a little **RITUAL.**

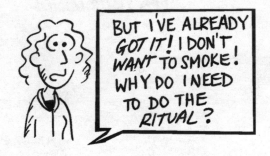

BUT I'VE ALREADY *GOT IT!* I DON'T *WANT* TO SMOKE! WHY DO I NEED TO DO THE *RITUAL?*

To signify your **LIBERTY**
but, more importantly,
to ensure that you have
the **CERTAINTY** to say:

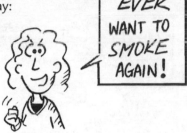

If you have not smoked for a few days – just confirm
that you have already smoked your **FINAL CIGARETTE**.
If you have been smoking while reading this book,
even if you have already **LOST ANY DESIRE** to smoke,
prove it to yourself through this ceremony.

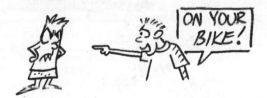

IT'S THE BIG GOODBYE.

SO HERE ARE YOUR FINAL INSTRUCTIONS FOR THE LAST CIGARETTE AND BEYOND:

1. Extinguish the final cigarette with a feeling of **ELATION**.

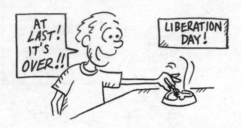

2. Be aware that the **LITTLE MONSTER** will be trying to **TRICK YOU**.

He'll moan...

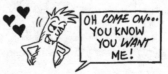

he'll flirt...

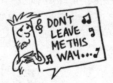

he'll pretend to be your **BEST BUDDY**.

It's like in those **THRILLER MOVIES**...

There's the heroine, safe inside her
house, while there's a **MONSTER**
outside, banging on the door.

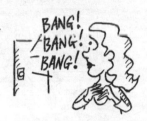

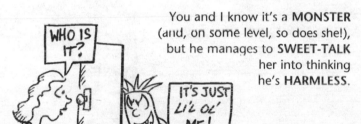

You and I know it's a **MONSTER**
(and, on some level, so does she!),
but he manages to **SWEET-TALK**
her into thinking
he's **HARMLESS**.

You're sitting there watching her start to **WAVER**
and, next thing, the stupid fool is heading for
the door...

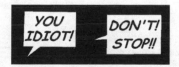

THE ILLUSTRATED <u>*Easyway*</u>

You can't believe she would even **CONSIDER** opening it. Doesn't she know he can **KILL** her?

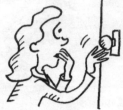

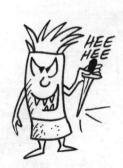

Well, *YOU* know better, don't you?

YOU MUST *NEVER, EVER* OPEN THAT DOOR!

3. DON'T AVOID SMOKERS OR SMOKING SITUATIONS.

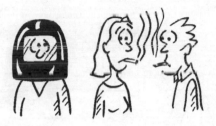

Go out and enjoy social occasions right from the start, even if you're surrounded by smokers. Realize you are not being **DEPRIVED – THEY ARE.**

4. DON'T ENVY SMOKERS.

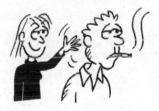

Why would you envy someone who is **TRAPPED?**

You know what? Deep down, they envy **YOU** because every one of them will be wishing they could be like you – **FREE FROM THE WHOLE FILTHY NIGHTMARE!**

5. REMEMBER, THERE IS NO SUCH THING AS 'JUST ONE' CIGARETTE

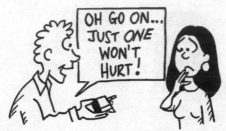

'Just one' cigarette is the first link in a whole **CHAIN OF MISERY**. If you light up 'just one', you just create a craving for another.

THAT CRAVING WILL NEVER BE SATISFIED!

Smoking is like **BASHING YOUR HEAD AGAINST A WALL** just to remind yourself how good it feels to **STOP**, or wearing **TIGHT SHOES** just to feel the relief of **TAKING THEM OFF**!

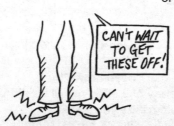

6. DON'T PUT OFF BECOMING A NON-SMOKER.

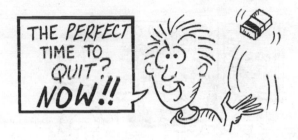

You become a non-smoker as soon as you cut off the **MONSTER'S SUPPLY.**

YOU ARE A NON-SMOKER FROM THE MOMENT YOU STUB OUT THE FINAL CIGARETTE!

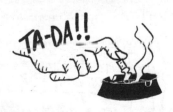

7. DON'T WORRY IF YOUR THOUGHTS CENTRE ON SMOKING FOR A WHILE.

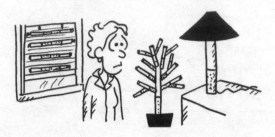

Why **WOULDN'T** they? A lot of your time
as a **SMOKER** was spent **THINKING** about **SMOKING**.
As a **NON-SMOKER**, you'll still **THINK** about it – after all,
it's been a **BIG PART** of your life until now.

The thing is, you'll be thinking **DIFFERENTLY**
about it, now.

THINK ABOUT IT, BUT
NEVER EVER
QUESTION YOUR DECISION.

Just hold **THIS** thought in your mind.

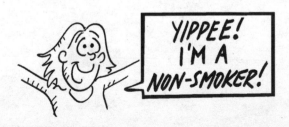

THE RITUAL

At last, it's time for the

CEREMONY OF THE LAST CIGARETTE.

LIGHT the last cigarette.

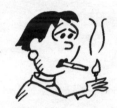

Feel it **BURNING** your **DELICATE LUNGS**.

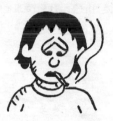

Feel how **PRECIOUS** and **VITAL** they are.

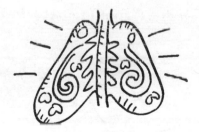

BREATHE IN THE SMOKE.

Experience the **TASTE** of the cigarette
in your mouth.

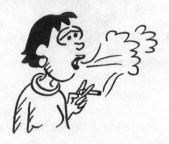

Notice how truly **FOUL** that cigarette tastes.

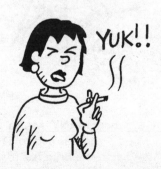

Now, shift your attention to your
BEAUTIFUL, FAITHFUL HEART.

Feel how it **RACES**.

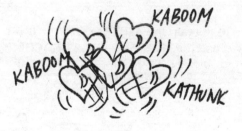

Think of how **MANY, MANY** times
your poor heart has had to **STRAIN**
like that as the drug has roared
through your **SYSTEM**.

Now, **STUB OUT** the cigarette
with a **FEELING OF ELATION**.

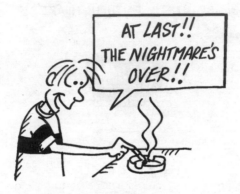

Gather up the **ASHTRAY** and the **BUTT**
and the **LIGHTER** and the **MATCHES**
and **ANYTHING** and **EVERYTHING**
to do with **SMOKING** and...

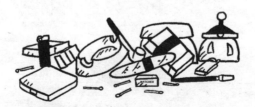

THROW THE WHOLE
MESS IN WITH THE TRASH!

You might feel like dancing around yelling:
'I'M FREE, I'M FREE!'

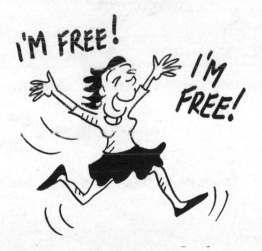

Now **STRIP** OFF those **STINKING CLOTHES**.

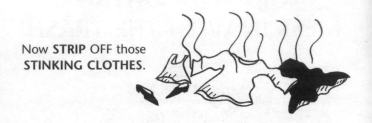

Take a **LONG, LUXURIOUS BATH**.

WASH YOUR HAIR.

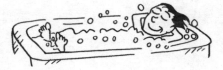

CLEAN YOUR TEETH.

SAVOUR how **CLEAN** and fresh you feel.

YOU'RE A HERO!

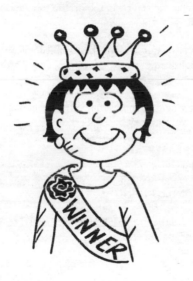

TELL ALLEN CARR'S EASYWAY
ORGANISATION THAT YOU'VE ESCAPED

Leave a comment on www.allencarr.com, like our Facebook page www.facebook.com/AllenCarr or write to the Worldwide Head Office address shown below.

ALLEN CARR'S EASYWAY CLINICS

The following list indicates the countries where Allen Carr's Easyway To Stop Smoking Clinics are currently operational. Check www.allencarr.com for latest additions to this list. The success rate at the clinics, based on the three month money-back guarantee, is over 90 per cent.

Selected clinics also offer sessions that deal with alcohol, other drugs, and weight issues. Please check with your nearest clinic for details.

Allen Carr's Easyway guarantees that you will find it easy to stop at the clinics or your money back.

ALLEN CARR'S EASYWAY

Worldwide Head Office
Park House, 14 Pepys Road, Raynes Park,
London SW20 8NH ENGLAND
Tel: +44 (0)208 9447761
Email: mail@allencarr.com
Website: www.allencarr.com

Worldwide Press Office
Tel: +44 (0)7970 88 44 52
Email: media@allencarr.com

UK Clinic Information and Central Booking Line
0800 389 2115 (Freephone)

UNITED KINGDOM	JAPAN
REPUBLIC OF IRELAND	LEBANON
AUSTRALIA	LITHUANIA
AUSTRIA	MAURITIUS
BELGIUM	MEXICO
BRAZIL	NETHERLANDS
BULGARIA	NEW ZEALAND
CANADA	NORWAY
CHILE	PERU
COLOMBIA	POLAND
CZECH REPUBLIC	PORTUGAL
DENMARK	ROMANIA
ESTONIA	RUSSIA
FINLAND	SERBIA
FRANCE	SINGAPORE
GERMANY	SLOVAKIA
GREECE	SLOVENIA
GUATEMALA	SOUTH AFRICA
HONG KONG	SOUTH KOREA
HUNGARY	SWEDEN
ICELAND	SWITZERLAND
INDIA	TURKEY
IRAN	UKRAINE
ISRAEL	UAE
ITALY	USA

Visit www.allencarr.com to access your nearest clinic's contact details.

OTHER ALLEN CARR PUBLICATIONS

Allen Carr's revolutionary Easyway method is available in a wide variety of formats, including digitally as audiobooks and ebooks, and has been successfully applied to a broad range of subjects.

For more information about Easyway publications, please visit **shop.allencarr.com**

Stop Smoking Now (with hypnotherapy CD)

Stop Smoking with Allen Carr (with 70-minute audio CD)

Your Personal Stop Smoking Plan

Finally Free!

The Easy Way for Women to Stop Smoking

The Illustrated Easy Way for Women to Stop Smoking

How to Be a Happy Non-Smoker

Smoking Sucks (Parent Guide with 16 page pull-out comic)

No More Ashtrays

The Little Book of Quitting

The Only Way to Stop Smoking Permanently

The Easy Way to Stop Smoking

How to Stop Your Child Smoking

The Easy Way to Control Alcohol

Your Personal Stop Drinking Plan

No More Hangovers

Lose Weight Now (with hypnotherapy CD)

No More Diets

The Easy Weigh to Lose Weight

Good Sugar Bad Sugar

The Easy Way to Quit Sugar

The Easy Way to Stop Gambling

No More Gambling (ebook)

No More Worrying

Allen Carr's Get Out of Debt Now

No More Debt (ebook)

The Easy Way to Enjoy Flying

No More Fear of Flying

Burning Ambition

Packing It In The Easy Way (the autobiography)

DISCOUNT VOUCHER FOR
ALLEN CARR'S EASYWAY CLINICS

Recover the price of this book when
you attend an
Allen Carr's Easyway Clinic
anywhere in the world.

Allen Carr has a global network
of clinics where he guarantees
you will find it easy to stop
smoking or your money back.

The success rate based on this
money-back guarantee is over 90 per cent.

When you book your appointment
mention this voucher and you will
receive a discount to the value
of this book. Contact your
nearest clinic for more information
on how the sessions work and
to book your appointment.
Not valid in conjunction with any other offer.